THE COMPLETE ANTI INFLAMMATORY DIET COOKBOOK FOR BEGINNERS 2024

Comprehensive Guide for Quick,easy and healthy recipes for immune boosting and reducing inflammation

Cristiana Castiglione

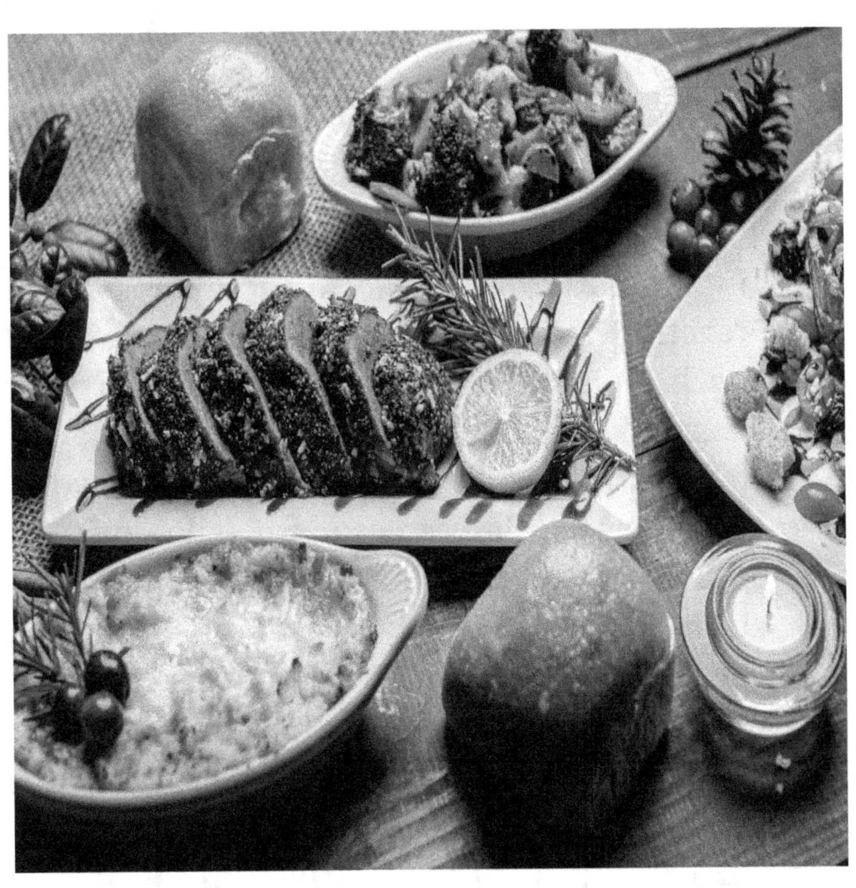

INTRODUCTION

UNDERSTANDING INFLAMMATION

What is inflammation?

inflammation is a basic and complex natural reaction that the body utilizes to safeguard itself from unsafe upgrades, like microbes, harmed cells, or aggravations. It is a pivotal piece of the body's invulnerable framework, intended to kill the reason for cell injury, get out harmed cells and tissues, and start tissue fixation. Basically, inflammation is a protection component that assumes a significant part in keeping up with the body's general wellbeing and respectability.

Component of inflammation

The course of inflammation includes a painstakingly coordinated succession of occasions. It regularly starts with the acknowledgment of unsafe improvements, which sets off a fountain of sub-atomic and cell reactions. The central participants in this cycle incorporate white platelets, safe cells, and flagging atoms like cytokines and chemokines. Veins likewise assume an imperative part by widening to increment bloodstream to the impacted region, prompting redness and warmth.

inflammation can be classified into two kinds: intense and constant. While chronic inflammation is a persistent, low-grade response that can contribute to various health issues, acute inflammation is a quick, short-term response that aims to eliminate the cause of cell injury.

Persistent inflammation
The Root Cause of Many Health Problems
While acute inflammation is a necessary and protective response, chronic inflammation can be harmful to the body. Constant inflammation is portrayed by a drawn out and supported fiery expression that can

endure for a really long time or even years. In contrast to acute inflammation, which is a process that is well-controlled and regulated, chronic inflammation has the potential to become dysregulated and contribute to the onset of a variety of health issues.

Medical problems Related with Constant inflammation:

1.   Autoimmune diseases: Constant aggravation is frequently connected to immune system problems, where the invulnerable framework erroneously goes after sound tissues and organs.

2.   Cardiovascular Diseases: Persevering inflammation can prompt the improvement of atherosclerosis, a condition where the veins become limited and solidified, expanding the gamble of respiratory failures and strokes.

3. Neurodegenerative Diseases: Constant inflammation has been ensnared in the movement of neurodegenerative circumstances like Alzheimer's and Parkinson's sickness.

4. Cancer: Fiery cycles can add to the commencement, advancement, and movement of disease by advancing the development and endurance of threatening cells.

5. Metabolic Disorders: Conditions like heftiness and type 2 diabetes are related with constant inflammation, which can add to insulin obstruction and metabolic brokenness.

In order to develop strategies for both preventing and managing a variety of health issues, it is essential to comprehend the causes and effects of chronic inflammation.

The Advantages of an Anti-Inflammatory Diet

Because chronic inflammation has such a significant negative impact on health, it is becoming increasingly recognized that following an anti-inflammatory diet is an effective strategy for enhancing one's overall well-being. An inflammation diet includes settling on food decisions that assist with diminishing inflammation in the body and advance a reasonable safe reaction.

Parts of a inflammation Diet:

1. Vegetables and Fruits: Plentiful in cell reinforcements, nutrients, and minerals, leafy foods assume an essential part in diminishing inflammation. These food

varieties give fundamental supplements that help the body's regular guard components.

2. Greasy Fish: Omega-3 unsaturated fats found in greasy fish like salmon and mackerel have calming properties. They are good for your heart and help keep the body's inflammatory response in check.

3. Entire Grains: Fiber and nutrients found in whole grains like quinoa and brown rice help maintain a healthy gut microbiome. Reduced inflammation is linked to a healthy gut microbiome.

4. Seeds and Nuts: Almonds, pecans, and flaxseeds are wealthy in omega-3 unsaturated fats and cell reinforcements, making them significant augmentations to an inflammation diet.

5. Spices and Spices: Turmeric, ginger, garlic, and different spices and flavors have inflammation and cancer prevention agent

properties. Incorporating these into one's diet may help to lessen inflammation.

Food varieties to Restrict or Stay away from:

1.   Handled Foods: Handled food sources frequently contain undesirable fats, refined sugars, and added substances that can advance aggravation. Restricting their utilization is fundamental for a calming diet.

2.   Sweet Beverages: Elevated degrees of added sugars in refreshments like soft drinks and caffeinated drinks are connected to aggravation and different metabolic issues. Picking water or natural teas is a better choice.

3.   Trans Fats: Trans fats, which can cause inflammation and are found in a lot of processed and fried foods, should be avoided in an anti-inflammatory diet.

4. Red Meat Excess: While lean wellsprings of protein are advantageous, extreme utilization of red meat, particularly handled meats, has been related with inflammation. Picking plant-based protein sources can be a better other option.

All in all, understanding aggravation is essential for keeping up with ideal wellbeing. While intense inflammation is a defensive reaction, constant inflammation can add to a scope of medical problems. Embracing an inflammation diet, wealthy in organic products, vegetables, greasy fish, entire grains, nuts, and seeds, while restricting handled food sources and unfortunate facts, is a functional and compelling method for supporting the body's normal protections and advance in general prosperity. The significance of lifestyle factors, including diet, in managing inflammation becomes increasingly apparent as research in this field continues to advance.

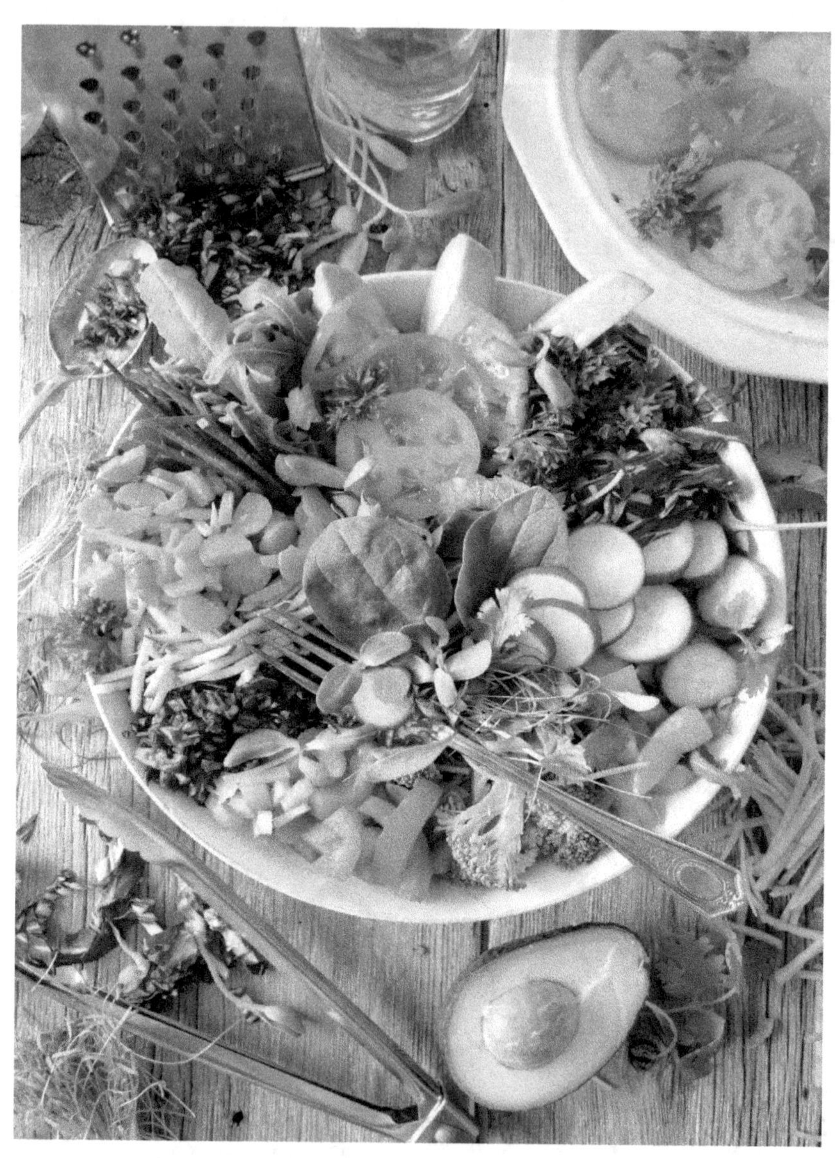

Chapter one

Getting Started

Key Standards of the inflammation Diet

Lately, there has been a developing familiarity with the effect of inflammation on generally speaking wellbeing. Ongoing inflammation is connected to different infections, including coronary illness, diabetes, and immune system problems. Thus, many individuals are going to inflammation consumes less calories as a proactive way to deal with advance prosperity and forestall medical problems.

Figuring out inflammation

Prior to diving into the critical standards of the inflammation diet, understanding inflammation is fundamental. inflammation is the body's normal reaction to injury or disease. However, numerous health issues can arise when inflammation becomes chronic. The calming diet means to moderate constant aggravation by advancing the utilization of food sources with inflammation properties and limiting those that add to inflammation.

Adjusting Omega-3 and Omega-6 Unsaturated fats

One central guideline of the calming diet is accomplishing a harmony between omega-3 and omega-6 unsaturated fats. The two kinds of unsaturated fats are fundamental for the body, however a lopsidedness, frequently brought about by a Western eating regimen high in handled food sources, can add to inflammation. Omega-3 unsaturated fats, tracked down in greasy fish, flaxseeds, and pecans, make calming impacts, while omega-6 unsaturated fats, predominant in vegetable oils and handled snacks, can be supportive of provocative when consumed in overabundance.

Emphasizing Whole Foods Whole, nutrient-dense foods are the foundation of the anti-inflammatory diet. Organic products, vegetables, entire grains, nuts, and seeds are wealthy in cancer prevention agents and phytochemicals that battle inflammation. These food sources additionally give fundamental nutrients and minerals that help generally speaking wellbeing. Picking entire food sources over handled choices lessens the admission of added substances and additives that might add to inflammation.

<u>Overseeing Glucose Levels</u>

Balancing out glucose levels is urgent for forestalling inflammation. Eating high-sugar and refined carb food sources can prompt spikes in glucose, setting off a fiery reaction. The inflammation diet advances complex starches, for example, entire grains and vegetables, which discharge glucose slowly, assisting with keeping up with consistent glucose levels.

Counting Calming Spices and Flavors

Spices and flavors have been utilized for quite a long time for flavor as well as for their restorative properties. Numerous spices and flavors show inflammation impacts. Turmeric, ginger, cinnamon, and garlic are remarkable models. These ingredients not only make food taste better but also have additional anti-inflammatory properties.

<u>Food varieties to Incorporate and Keep away from</u>

<u>Food varieties to Incorporate</u>

<u>Greasy Fish</u>

Greasy fish, like salmon, mackerel, and sardines, are wealthy in omega-3 unsaturated fats. These fundamental fats make strong calming impacts, assisting with decreasing inflammation at the cell level. Remembering greasy fish for the eating routine no less than two times every week is a foundation of the inflammation approach.

<u>Leafy Greens</u>

Leafy greens like Swiss chard, kale, and spinach are loaded with antioxidants, vitamins, and minerals. Inflammation can be reduced by neutralizing free radicals in the body with these nutrients. Integrating various mixed greens into servings of mixed greens, smoothies, or cooked dishes is a straightforward yet compelling method for helping calming admission.

Berries

Berries, like blueberries, strawberries, and raspberries, are stacked with cell reinforcements known as flavonoids. These mixtures have inflammation properties and may assist with diminishing the gamble of persistent infections. Berries can be delighted in new, added to yogurt, or mixed into smoothies for a tasty and stimulating treat.

Nuts and Seeds

Almonds, pecans, flaxseeds, and chia seeds are amazing wellsprings of omega-3 unsaturated fats, fiber, and cancer prevention agents. These nuts and seeds add to heart wellbeing and have calming properties. Nibbling on a modest bunch of nuts or integrating them into dinners increases the value of the inflammation diet.

Olive Oil

Additional virgin olive oil is a staple in the Mediterranean eating regimen, famous for its inflammation impacts. It has polyphenols and monounsaturated fats that help reduce inflammation. Involving olive oil as the essential cooking oil or showering it over plates of mixed greens and vegetables is a basic method for improving the inflammation profile of feasts.

Turmeric

Curcumin, a potent anti-inflammatory compound, can be found in turmeric, a golden spice that is frequently used in curries. Adding turmeric to soups, stews, or pan-sears gives a warm flavor while giving inflammation benefits. Matching turmeric with dark pepper upgrades the assimilation of curcumin in the body.

Food varieties to Keep away from

Handled Food varieties

Handled food varieties, including inexpensive food, sweet bites, and accommodation feasts, frequently contain unfortunate fats, refined sugars, and added substances. These fixings can add to inflammation and subvert the advantages of a calming diet. Settling on entire, natural food varieties is fundamental for lessening fiery triggers.

Refined Carbs

White bread, cakes, and other refined carbs can cause fast spikes in glucose levels, advancing aggravation. Picking entire grains like quinoa, earthy colored rice, and oats gives supported energy without the adverse consequence on glucose.

Inordinate Red Meat

While lean wellsprings of red meat can be essential for a decent eating regimen, extreme utilization might add to inflammation. Handled and restored meats, like wieners and bacon, frequently contain added substances that can set off inflammation. Counting plant-based protein sources like beans and lentils can be a better other option.

High Sugar Admission

An eating routine high in added sugars is related to weight, diabetes, and inflammation. To lessen the inflammatory load, sugary beverages, sweets, and desserts should be limited. Anti-inflammatory principles are reflected in the choice of fresh fruit as a sweet treat or natural sweeteners like honey.

<u>Trans Fats</u>

Trans fats, frequently tracked down into to some degree hydrogenated oils, are known to advance aggravation and increment the gamble of coronary illness. An anti-inflammatory diet necessitates avoiding fried foods, margarine, and commercially baked goods that contain trans fats.

In rundown, the calming diet is a comprehensive way to deal with advancing wellbeing and forestalling constant sicknesses. By zeroing in on key standards, for example, adjusting unsaturated fats, stressing entire food varieties, overseeing glucose levels, and consolidating inflammation spices and flavors, people can make a supplement thick and inflammation battling eating plan. Picking various food varieties, including greasy fish, salad greens, berries, nuts, and olive oil, while staying away from handled food varieties, refined starches, over the top red meat, high sugar consumption, and trans fats, frames the groundwork of a calming way of life. Rolling out these dietary improvements can add to generally speaking prosperity and decrease the gamble of inflammation related medical problems.

Chapter Two

Constructing Your Kitchen to Reduce Inflammation

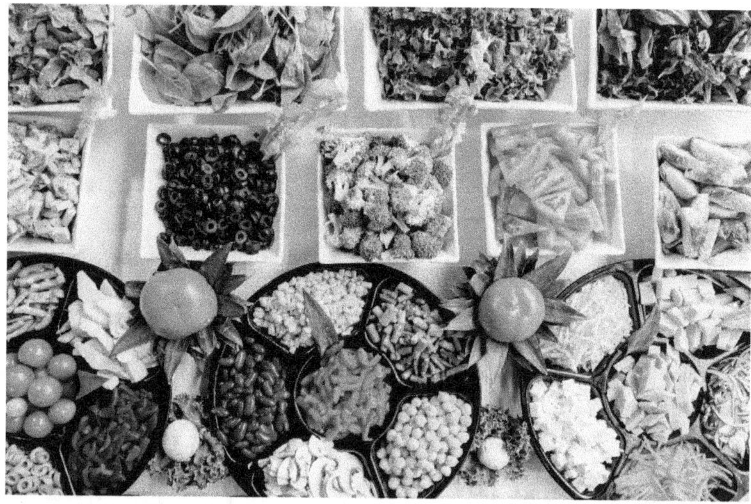

Certainly! A calming diet is centered around consolidating food sources that assist with diminishing irritation in the body, which is related with different ongoing illnesses. How about we examine the fundamental fixings and spices/flavors with calming properties exhaustively:

First, the Essentials:

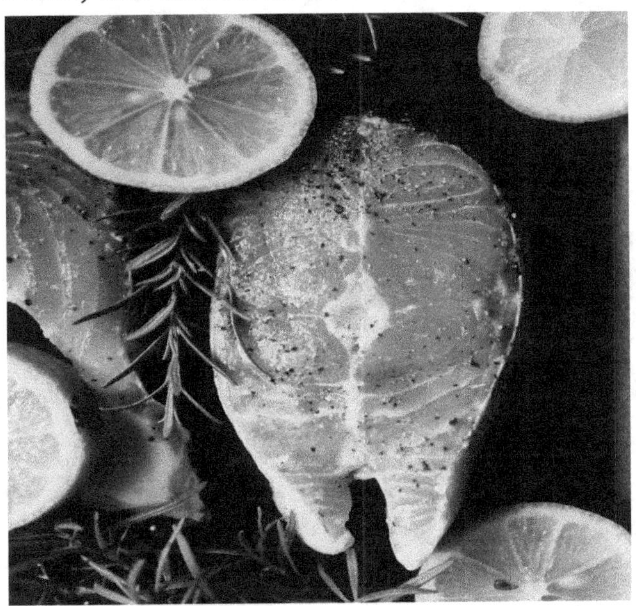

a) Crunchy Fish:
    - Wealthy in omega-3 unsaturated fats, especially EPA and DHA.
    - Tracked down in salmon, mackerel, sardines, and trout.
    - Omega-3s are known for their strong calming impacts.

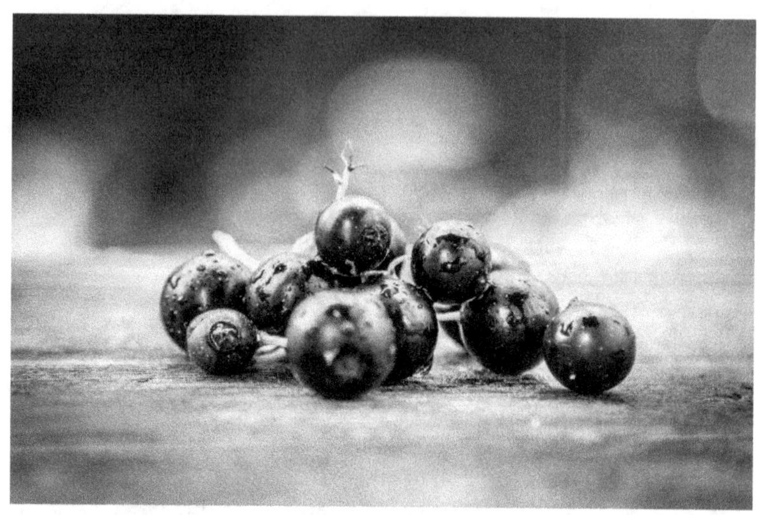

b]Berries:

- Blueberries, strawberries, raspberries, and blackberries.

- High in cell reinforcements, nutrients, and fiber.

- Battle oxidative pressure and irritation.

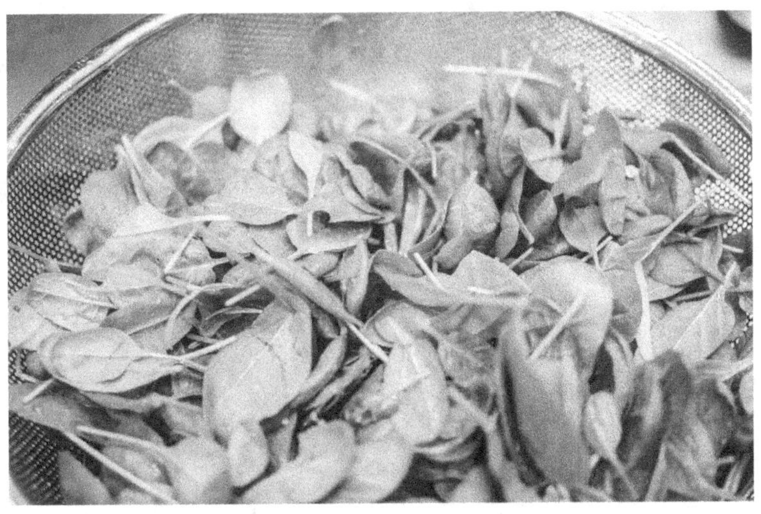

c) Verdant Greens:

- Swiss chard, collard greens, spinach, and kale

- Loaded with nutrients, minerals, and cell reinforcements.

- Assist with controlling the incendiary reaction.

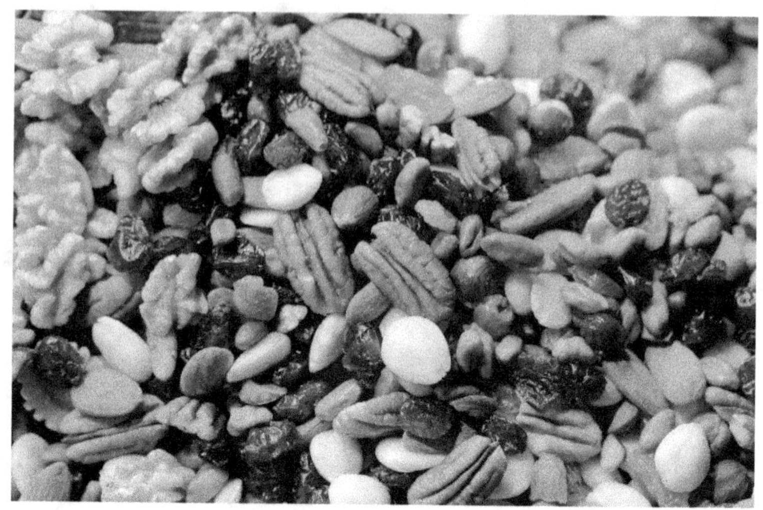

d) Seeds and Nuts: - Almonds, pecans, chia seeds, and flaxseeds.

- Supply antioxidants, fiber, and healthy fats.

For instance, almonds contain a lot of vitamin E and monounsaturated fats.

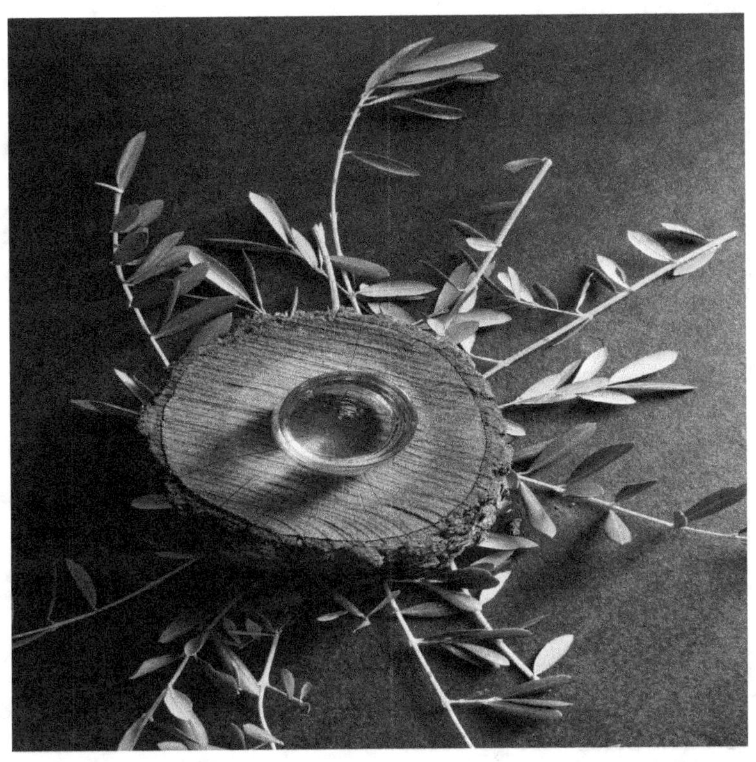

e) Olive Oil:

Olive oil that is extra-virgin is a crucial component.

- Contains oleocanthal, a calming compound.

- Replaces immersed fats with heart-solid monounsaturated fats.

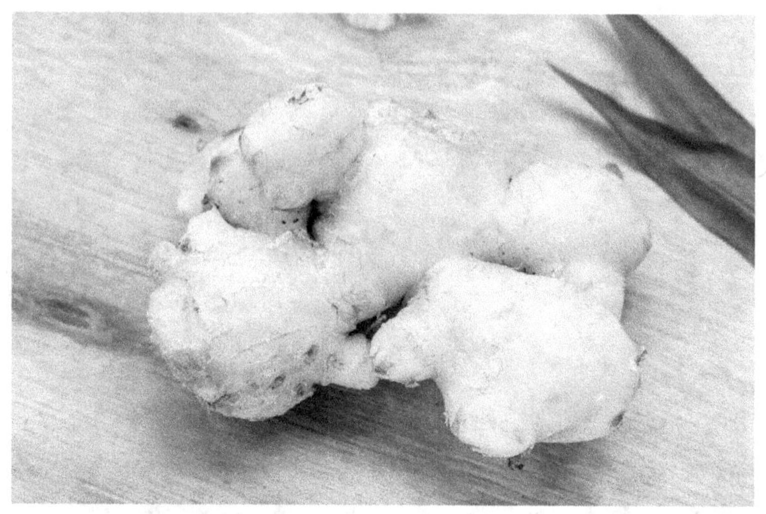

f) Ginger:

- Contains curcumin, a strong calming compound.

- Utilized for its therapeutic properties in traditional medicine.

- Frequently joined with dark pepper to upgrade retention.

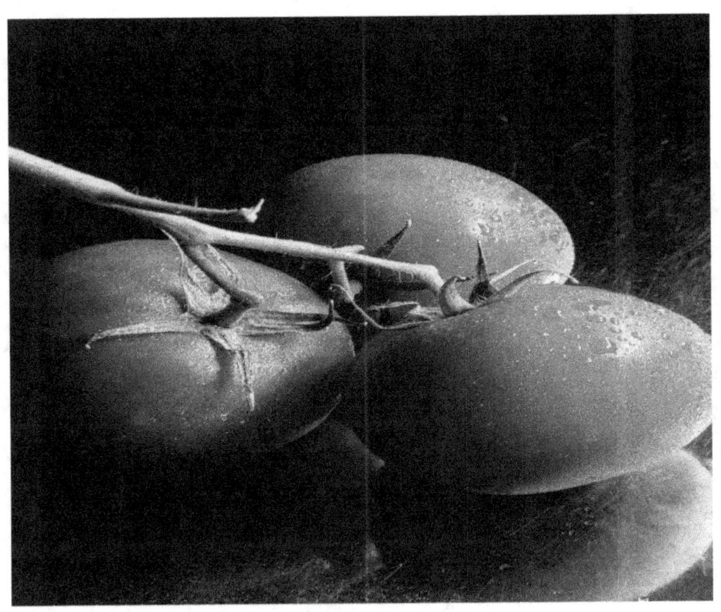

g):Tomatoes,

- Wealthy in lycopene, a cancer prevention agent with calming impacts.

- Cooking tomatoes can increase lycopene retention.

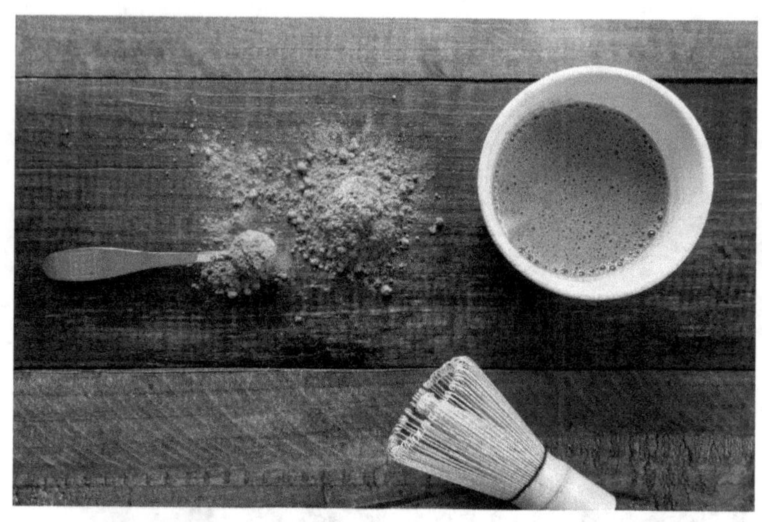

h) Green Tea:

- Has polyphenols in it, especially catechins.

- Known for their antioxidant and anti-inflammatory qualities.

- Supports diminishing irritation and forestalling cell harm

<u>**Herbs and spices that reduce inflammation:**</u>

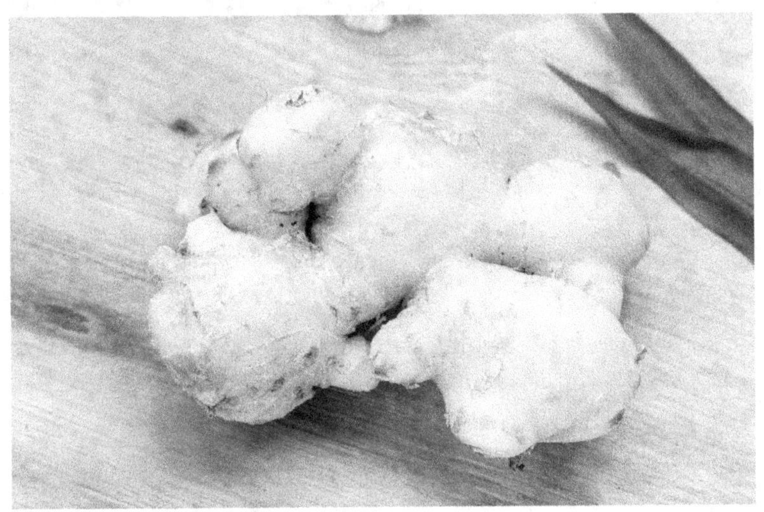

a) Ginger:

- Gingerol, which is known for its antioxidant and anti-inflammatory properties, is present.

- Utilized in different structures, for example, new, powdered, or as a tea.

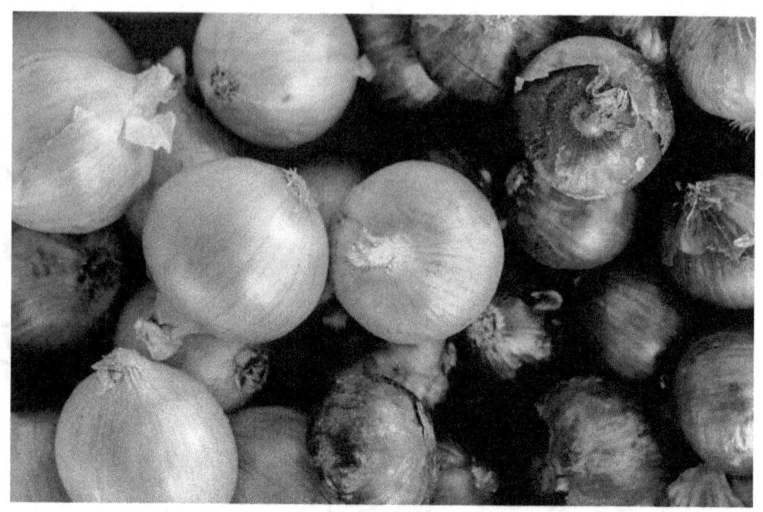

b) Onion:

- Allicin, a sulfur-containing compound, adds to its mitigating properties.

- Likewise has safe supporting advantages.

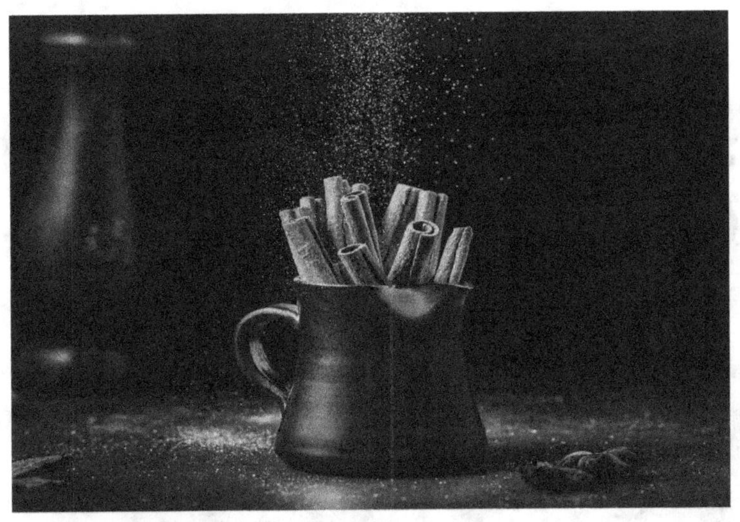

c) Cinnamon:

- Contains cell reinforcements with calming impacts.

- Aids in the regulation of blood sugar levels and reduces insulin resistance-associated inflammation.

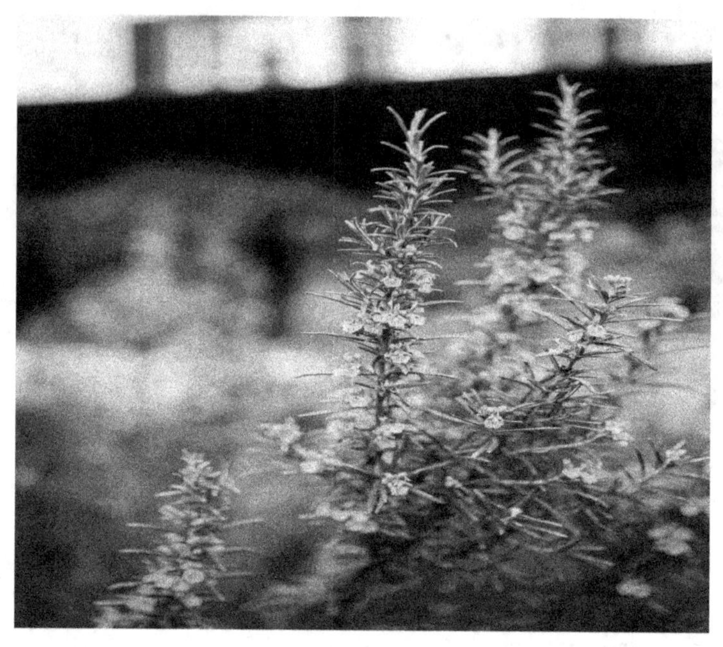

d) Rosemary:

- Contains compounds with anti-inflammatory properties, including rosmarinic acid.

- Adds flavor to dishes while giving medical advantages.

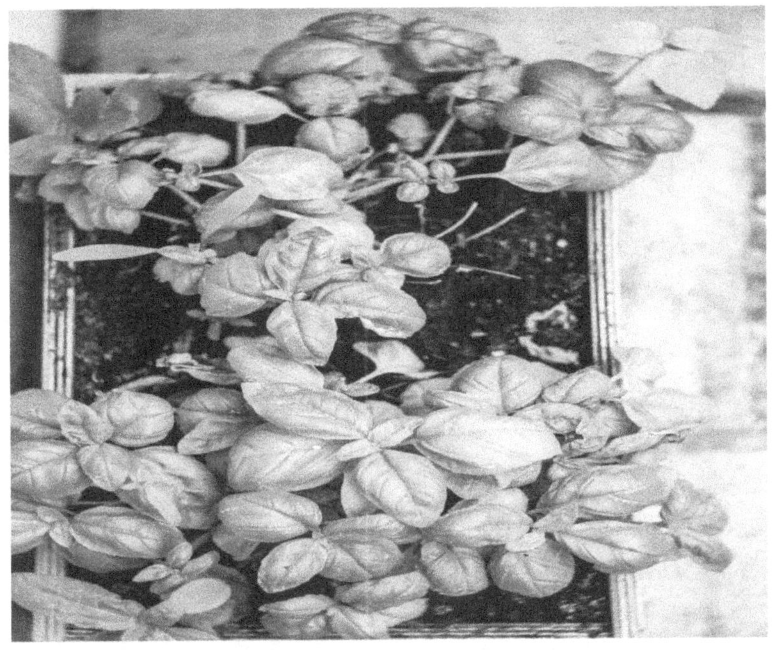

e) Basil:

- Wealthy in flavonoids, which make mitigating impacts.

- Improves the kind of different dishes.

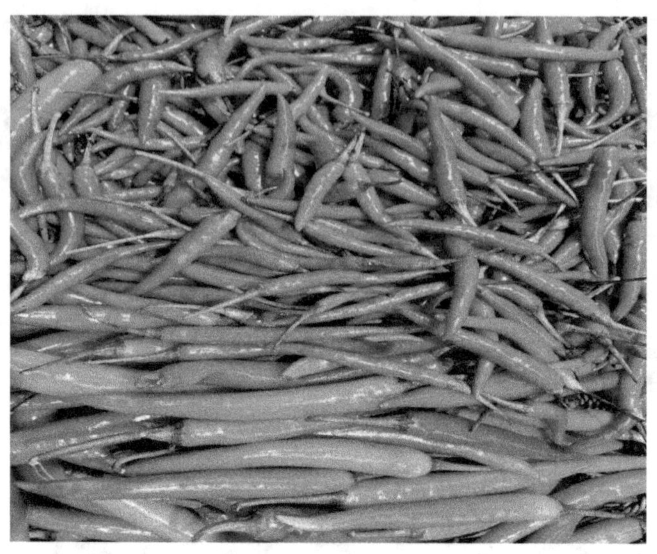

f) Cayenne Pepper:

The active ingredient, capsaicin, has anti-inflammatory properties.

- Additionally advances blood flow and may help with relief from discomfort.

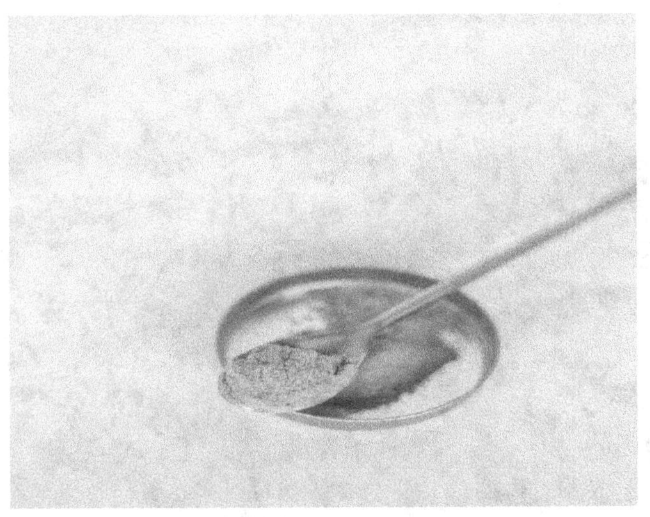

g) Turmeric:

- As well as being a fundamental fixing, turmeric is a strong calming zest.

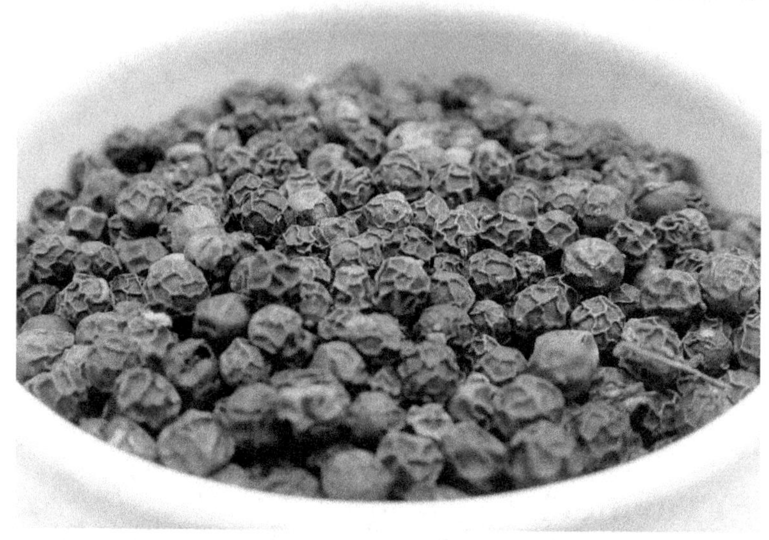

h) Dark Pepper:
   - Contains piperine, improving the assimilation of curcumin from turmeric.

Taking on a mitigating diet that incorporates these fundamental fixings and spices/flavors can add to generally speaking wellbeing and may help in overseeing irritation related conditions. Adjusting the admission of these food varieties as a component of a balanced and various diet is fundamental. Before making major changes to your diet, you should always talk to a doctor or a nutritionist, especially if you already have health problems.

Creating an Anti-Inflammatory Kitchen: Equipping, Cooking Utensils, and Cookware

How to Make Your Kitchen Anti-Inflammatory: Setting Up Cookware, Utensils, and Equipment In light of its potential health benefits, the significance of an anti-inflammatory diet has received a lot of attention in recent years. Ongoing aggravation is connected to different medical problems, including coronary illness, diabetes, and immune system issues. When you follow an anti-inflammatory diet, you have to be careful about what you eat, but it's just as important to think about the tools and equipment in your kitchen. In this thorough aide, we'll investigate how to prepare your kitchen, fundamental cooking tools, and the right cookware to help a calming way of life.

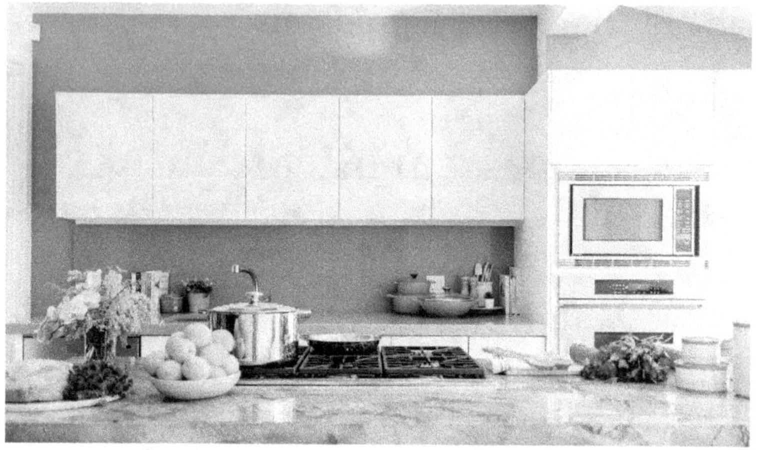

1) Preparing Your Kitchen:

a) Loading Up on Mitigating Fixings:

The underpinning of a calming kitchen starts with the fixings you use. Focus on entire food sources like natural products, vegetables, lean proteins, and sound fats. Include a variety of vibrant fruits and vegetables that are high in antioxidants and aid in reducing inflammation. Include omega-3 fatty acids from flaxseeds, walnuts, and fatty fish. Whole grains have more nutrients and fiber than refined grains.

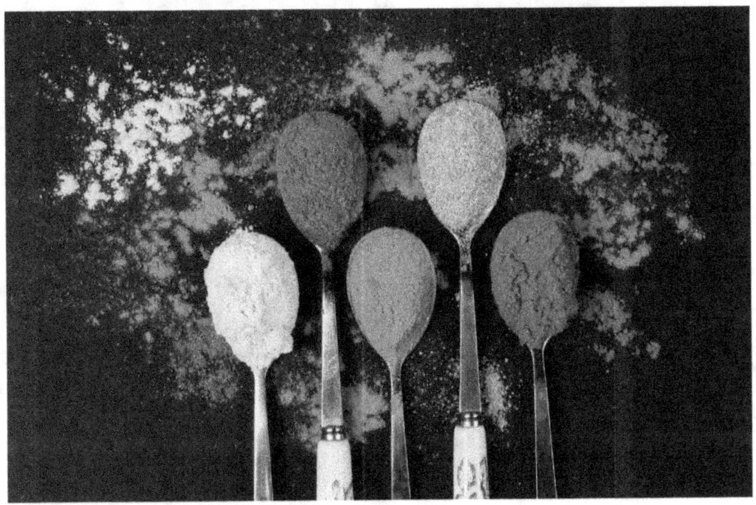

b) Spices and Flavors:

Spices and flavors add flavor to your dishes as well as bring calming properties. Turmeric, ginger, garlic, cinnamon, and cayenne pepper are pantry staples. These fixings contain bioactive mixtures that have been displayed to lessen aggravation and advance generally wellbeing.

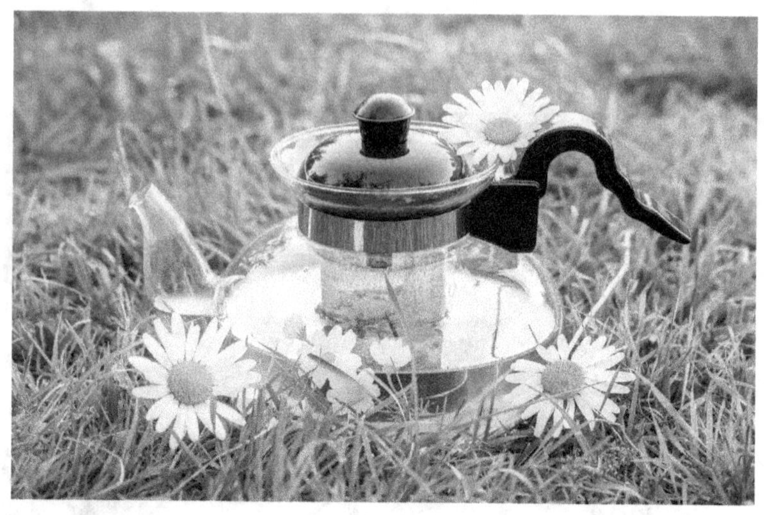

c) Beneficial Oils:

Maintaining an anti-inflammatory kitchen requires choosing the right cooking oils. Choose oils with a high smoke point, like avocado oil or extra virgin olive oil. These oils are wealthy in monounsaturated fats and have calming properties. Stay away from oils high in omega-6 unsaturated fats, similar to vegetable and soybean oil, as a lopsidedness of omega-3 to omega-6 proportions can add to aggravation.

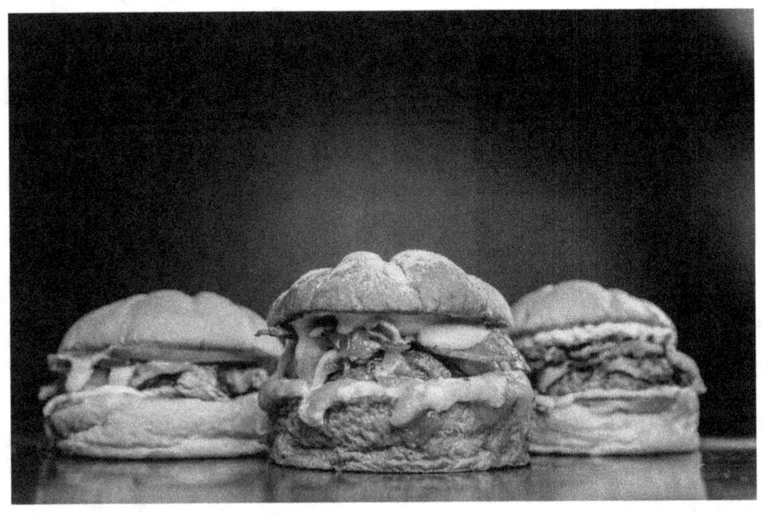

d) Limiting Handled Food varieties:

Remove processed and refined foods from your kitchen because they frequently contain additives, preservatives, and unhealthy fats that can exacerbate inflammation. Nuts, seeds, and fresh fruits are good alternatives to processed snacks.

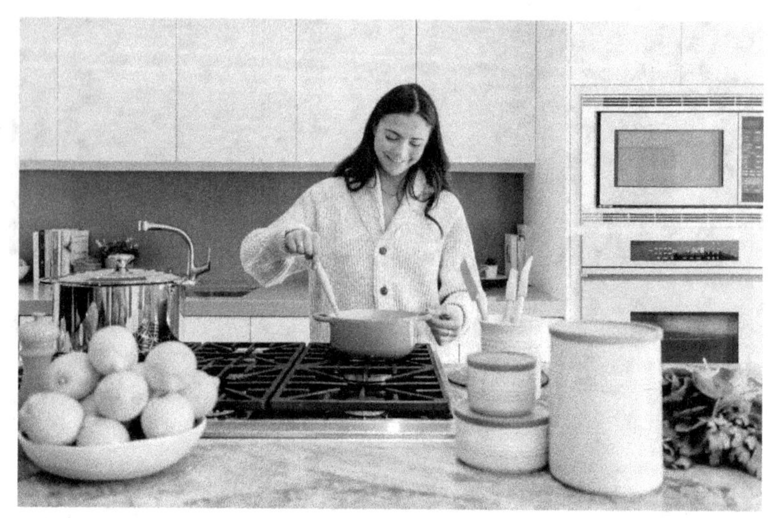

Essential Cooking Tools:

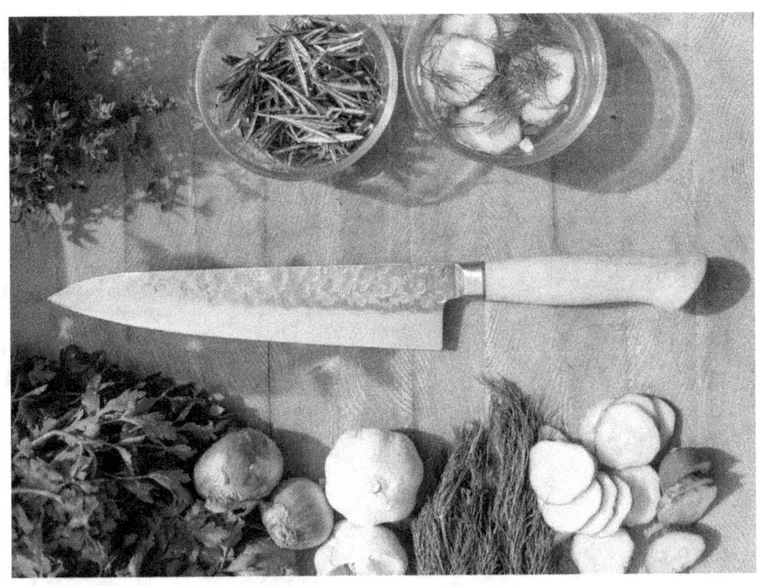

a) Knives of High Quality:

Putting resources into excellent blades is fundamental for setting up various new natural products, vegetables, and lean proteins. Dull blades can prompt wasteful cleaving and may bring about lopsided cooking. Keep your blades sharp to make dinner planning more pleasant and effective.

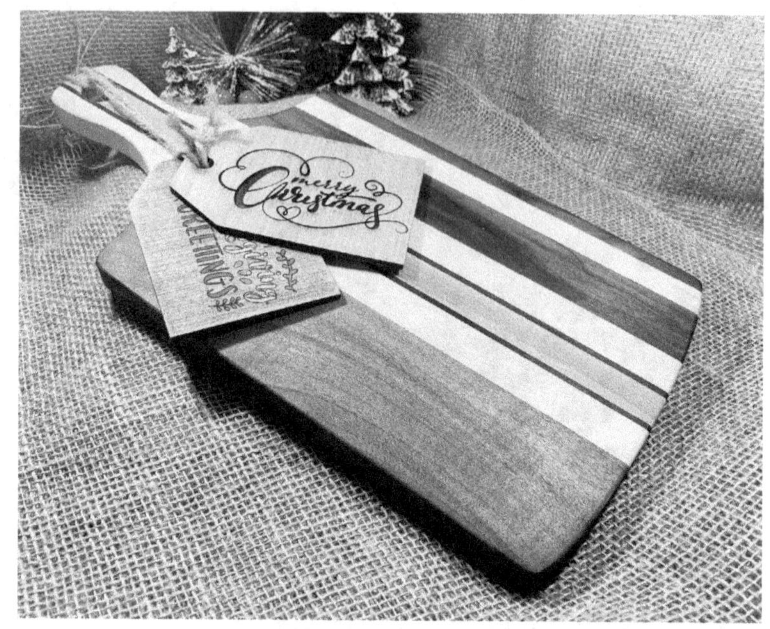

b) Cutting Sheets:

Pick cutting sheets made of materials that are not difficult to clean and keep up with, for example, bamboo or sans bpa plastic. Having separate cutting sheets for meat, poultry, and vegetables forestalls cross-tainting, guaranteeing the security of your feasts.

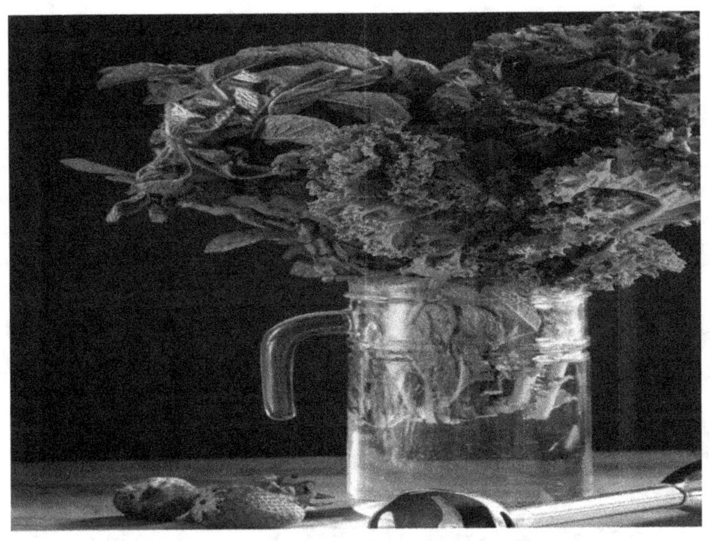

c) Food Processor or Blender:

A food processor or blender is a flexible instrument for making smoothies, soups, sauces, and plunges. Consolidate calming fixings like berries, salad greens, and nuts to get ready to supplement thick and aggravation battling recipes.

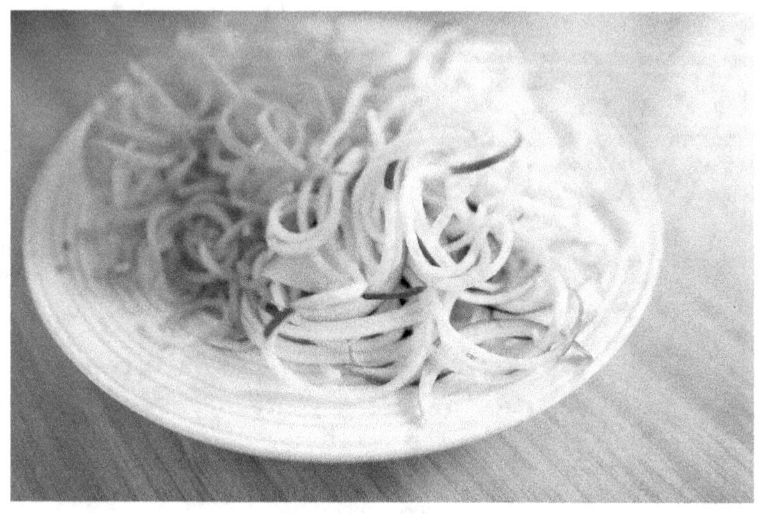

d) Vegetable Spiralizer:

A vegetable spiralizer is a tomfoolery and imaginative method for integrating more vegetables into your feasts. Use it to make zucchini noodles or spiralized yams as a nutritious option in contrast to conventional pasta.

e) Microplane Grater:

A microplane grater is ideal for adding zing to your dishes. Use it to grind ginger, garlic, or citrus strips to mix your feasts with flavor and mitigating compounds.

f) Lemon Squeezer:

New citrus juice is an extraordinary method for upgrading the flavor of your dishes without adding undesirable fixings. Using a lemon squeezer, you can easily extract juice and incorporate it into beverages, marinades, and dressings.

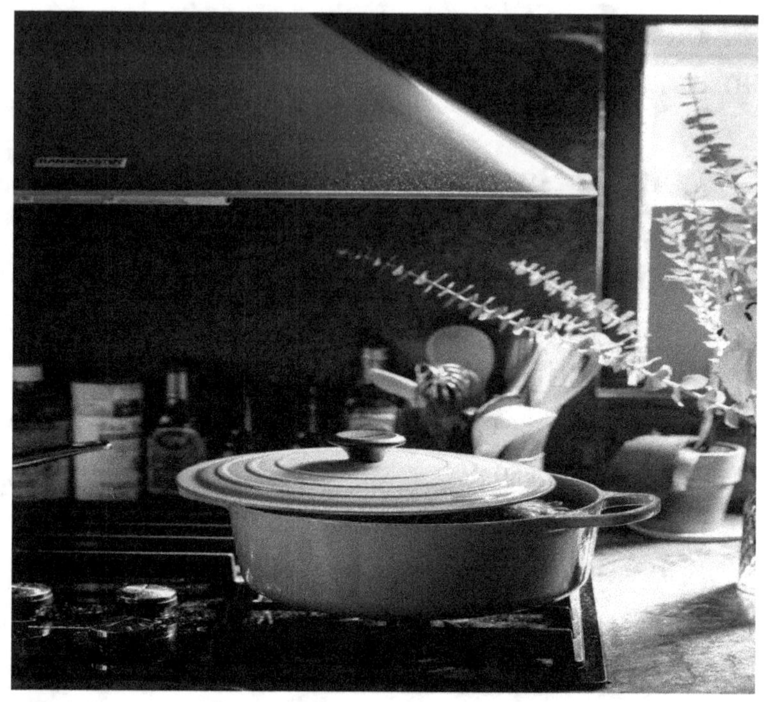

<u>**Selecting the Best Cookware:**</u>

a) Cookware With No Sticks:

Choose nonstick cookware coated with ceramic or PTFE-free materials. This diminishes the requirement for unreasonable preparation oils and keeps food from staying, advancing a better cooking process.

b) Treated Steel:

Treated steel cookware is strong, impervious to rust and consumption, and doesn't filter hurtful synthetic compounds into your food. It's a protected and flexible choice for different cooking strategies, including sautéing and bubbling.

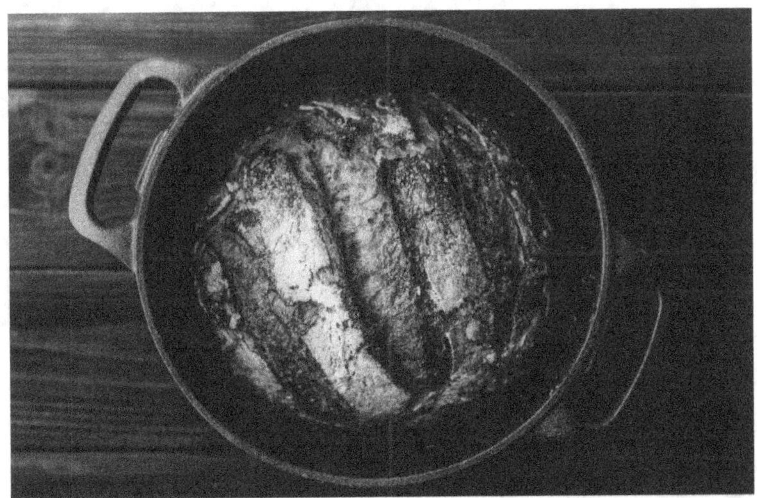

c) Cast Iron:

Project iron cookware is known for its in any event, warming and superb intensity maintenance. Cooking with cast iron likewise adds a limited quantity of iron to your food, which can be valuable for those with a lack of iron. Be that as it may, be aware of keeping up with and preparing cast iron appropriately to forestall rust.

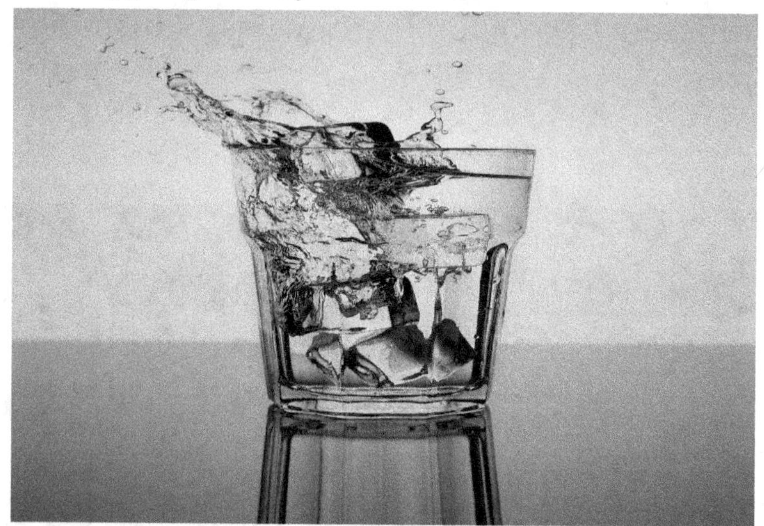

d) Glass:

Cookware made of glass is a safe choice for baking and roasting. It ensures that your meals do not contain any harmful substances because it does not leach any chemicals into them. Glass also makes it simple to monitor your cooking process.

e) Keeping away from Teflon and Aluminum:

Teflon-covered cookware and aluminum skillet ought to be stayed away from, particularly when scratched or harmed. Teflon can deliver poisonous exhaust when overheated, and aluminum has been related with neurological issues. Supplant these with more secure options like treated steel or artistic covered cookware.

Beyond what you cook, creating an anti-inflammatory kitchen is about more than just that; It includes the equipment and tools you use. Outfitting your kitchen with the right fixings, cooking tools, and cookware makes way for a better and more irritation accommodating way of life. By settling on smart decisions in your kitchen, you can improve the calming advantages of your eating routine and add to general prosperity.

Chapter Three

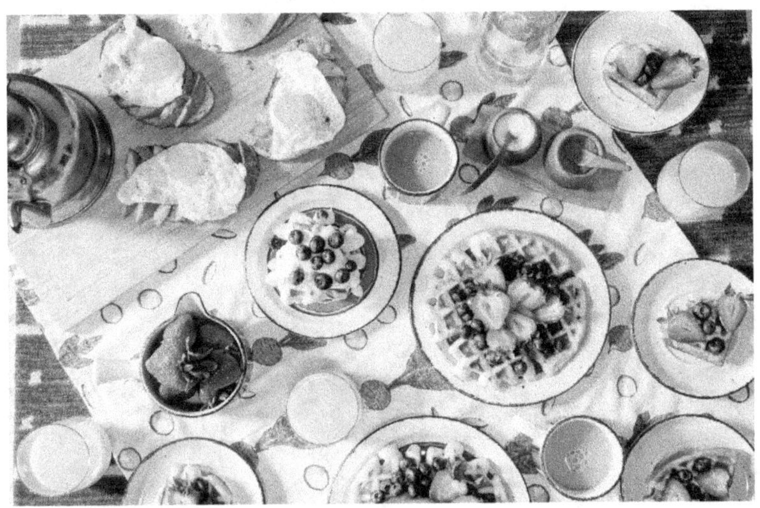

<u>Yummy and Packed with Nutrients Recipes</u>

Certainly! A mitigating diet centers around decreasing irritation in the body by underlining food sources that have calming properties. Here is an escalated conversation on breakfast choices inside a calming diet:

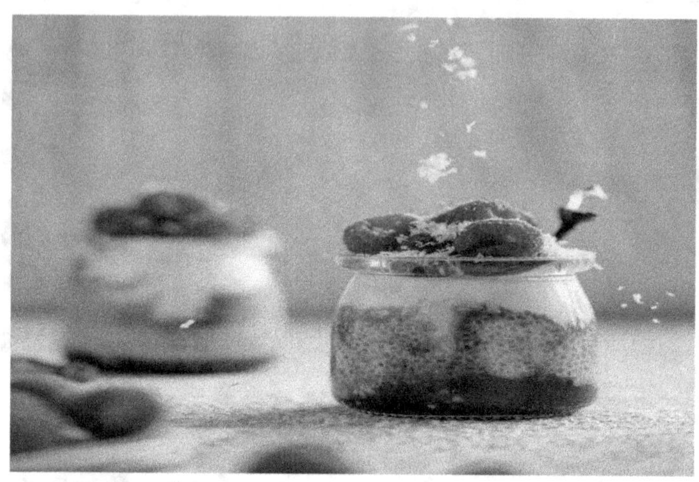

a. Chia Seed Pudding:

- Chia seeds are wealthy in omega-3 unsaturated fats, which make mitigating impacts.

- Join chia seeds with almond milk, berries, and a dash of honey for a delectable and nutritious breakfast.

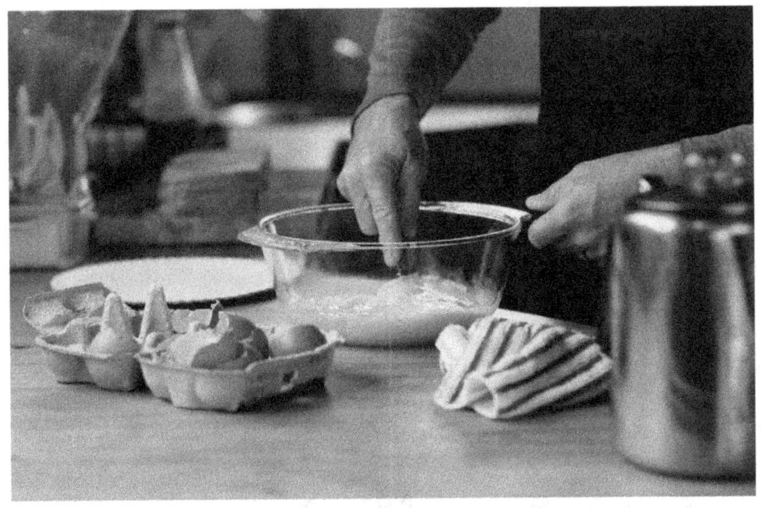

b. "Turmeric Scrambled Eggs":

- Turmeric contains curcumin, a powerful mitigating compound. Adding it to fried eggs supports their calming properties.

- Consolidate vegetables like spinach and tomatoes for added supplements.

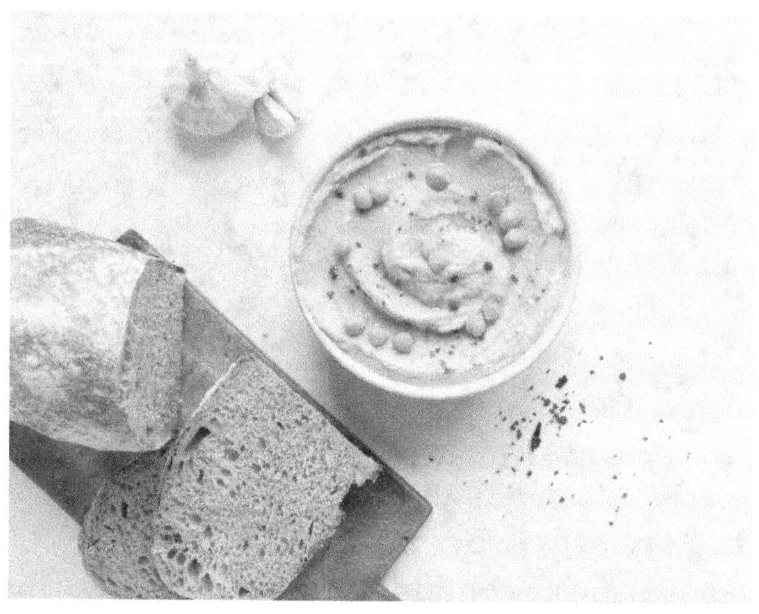

c. Avocado Toast with Entire Grain Bread:

- Avocado is loaded with monounsaturated fats and cell reinforcements, adding to a calming diet.

- Pick entire grain bread for fiber, supporting stomach wellbeing and decreasing aggravation.

d. Omelet with Salmon and Vegetables:

- Greasy fish like salmon contain omega-3s, known for their calming benefits.

- Incorporate vivid vegetables like chime peppers and spinach for extra cell reinforcements.

e. Quinoa Breakfast Bowl:

- Quinoa is a finished protein and contains different calming compounds.

- Blend cooked quinoa with new organic products, nuts, and a shower of honey for a delightful and calming breakfast.

<u>**Bowls of energizing smoothies**</u>:

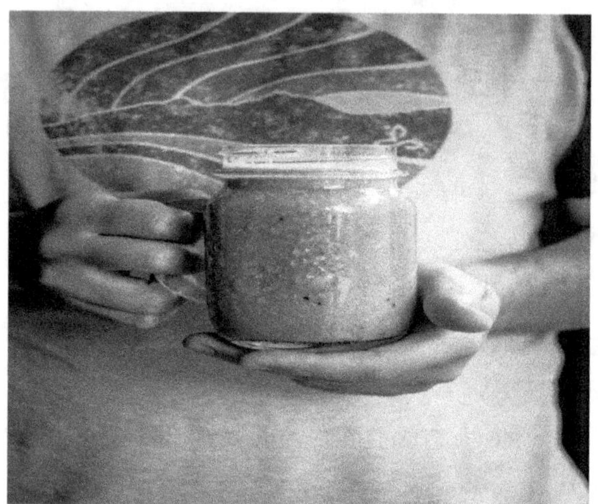

a. Bowl for Green Smoothie: In a smoothie, spinach, kale, and other leafy greens provide antioxidants and nutrients that reduce inflammation.

- Add organic products like pineapple and mango for pleasantness and additional nutrients.

b. Smoothie Bowl with Turmeric and Berries:

- Berries are wealthy in cell reinforcements, and turmeric adds a strong calming punch.

- For creaminess and additional protein, blend with Greek yogurt or a plant-based alternative.

c. Papaya and Ginger Smoothie Bowl:

Ginger has been shown to have anti-inflammatory effects, and papaya contains enzymes with anti-inflammatory properties.

- Top with seeds and a base like coconut milk for extra texture.

<u>Varieties of Anti-Inflammatory Oatmeal:</u>

a. Turmeric and Cinnamon Oatmeal:

- Turmeric and cinnamon both have mitigating properties.

Oats should be cooked with a pinch of cinnamon and turmeric before being topped with fresh fruits and nuts.

b.Berries and Almond Spread Oatmeal:

Almond butter contains healthy fats and berries are high in antioxidants.

- Blend into oats for a scrumptious and mitigating breakfast.

c. Overnight Oats with Golden Milk:

- Brilliant milk, made with turmeric and different flavors, is a conventional calming drink.

- Consolidate these flavors with oats, chia seeds, and your decision of milk for a helpful and nutritious short-term choice.

In synopsis, a morning meal zeroed in on a mitigating diet incorporates fixings like greasy fish, mixed greens, berries, nuts, seeds, and flavors like turmeric and ginger.

These fixings not just give a delectable beginning to the day yet in addition add to decreasing irritation in the body and advancing in general wellbeing.

Bright Lunch Ideas

a. Grilled Salmon with Quinoa and Simmered Vegetables:
- Salmon furnishes omega-3 unsaturated fats with mitigating impacts.
- Quinoa adds protein and fiber, while different simmered vegetables offer a range of supplements and cell reinforcements.

b. Wraps with Chickpea and Turmeric Salad:
Chickpeas are a great source of protein and fiber from plants.
- Blend chickpeas in with turmeric, olive oil, and different beautiful veggies. Serve in

entire grain wraps for a delightful and calming lunch.

c. Miso-Coated Tofu Mix Fry:

- Tofu is wealthy in protein and low in immersed fat, advancing a calming diet.

- Pan sear tofu with beautiful vegetables and a miso-based sauce for a delightful and wellbeing stuffed lunch.

d. Quinoa and Vegetable Buddha Bowl:

- Make a bowl with a base of quinoa, finished off with different vivid vegetables, for example, ringer peppers, carrots, and cherry tomatoes.

- Shower with olive oil and a sprinkle of spices for added calming benefits.

e. Lentil and Vegetable Stuffed Ringer Peppers:

- Lentils are high in fiber and protein, making them a phenomenal expansion to a calming lunch.

- Stuff chime peppers with a combination of lentils, tomatoes, and spices, then prepare for a beautiful and nutritious dinner.

Combinations of colorful salads:

a. Kale and Berry Salad:
- Kale is a supplement force to be reckoned with, and berries carry cell reinforcements to the blend.

- For a vibrant and anti-inflammatory salad, toss kale with a variety of berries, walnuts, and balsamic vinaigrette.

b. Rainbow Quinoa Salad:
- Quinoa fills in as a protein-pressed base for this serving of mixed greens.

- Add bright vegetables like cherry tomatoes, cucumbers, and ringer peppers. For a refreshing anti-inflammatory option, top with a dressing with a citrus flavor.

c. Salad with Avocado and Citrus:
   - Avocado gives solid fats, and citrus organic products bring L-ascorbic acid and cell reinforcements.
   - For a delicious and anti-inflammatory salad, combine them with mixed greens, red onions, and a light olive oil dressing.

 d. Mango and Dark Bean Salad:
   Black beans provide protein and fiber, while mangoes provide the natural sweetness.
   - Blend in with red onions, cilantro, and a lime-based dressing for a tropical and calming salad.

e. Greek Salad topped with Salmon:
   A classic Greek salad gets its omega-3 fatty acids from salmon.
   - Include colorful vegetables like red onions, cherry tomatoes, and cucumbers. A dish that is anti-inflammatory and takes its cues from the Mediterranean can be dressed with olive oil and oregano.

<u>Delicious Stews and Soups:</u>

a. "Turmeric Lentil Soup":

Lentils are a good source of protein and fiber from plants.

- Inject the soup with turmeric, garlic, and ginger for a delightful and mitigating choice.

b. Stew with Chickpeas and Vegetables:

- Chickpeas offer protein and fiber, while various vegetables contribute nutrients and minerals.

- Prepare a broth rich in anti-inflammatory herbs like rosemary and thyme before cooking.

c. Soup with Spinach and Quinoa:

- Spinach gives iron and cancer prevention agents, and quinoa adds protein.

By combining these with tomatoes, herbs, and vegetable broth, you can make a nutritious soup.

d. Sweet Potato and Ginger Bisque:
   - Yams are wealthy in beta-carotene and have mitigating properties.
   - Mix cooked yams with ginger and vegetable stock for a rich and calming soup.

e. Chickpea and Tomato Basil Stew:
   - Tomatoes are high in lycopene, known for its enemy of a filling stew. Add a sprinkle of olive oil and season with mitigating flavors like turmeric and cumin to upgrade the flavor profile while expanding medical advantages.

<u>Ways to upgrade Mitigating Dinners:</u>

1. Include beneficial fats:
   - Utilize olive oil, avocado, and nuts to add monounsaturated fats and omega-3 unsaturated fats, which add to decreasing aggravation.

2. Pick Beautiful Vegetables:

- Various tones in vegetables demonstrate an assortment of phytonutrients. Go for the gold of varieties in your dinners to guarantee a different scope of calming compounds.

3. Choose Entire Grains:

- Entire grains like quinoa, earthy colored rice, and oats are wealthy in fiber and add to destroy wellbeing, which is firmly connected to aggravation guidelines.

4. Incorporate Lean Proteins:

- Integrate wellsprings of lean protein like fish, tofu, vegetables, and poultry to help muscle wellbeing and decrease irritation.

5. Utilize Mitigating Spices and Spices:

The anti-inflammatory properties of turmeric, ginger, garlic, cinnamon, and other ingredients are well-known. Put a lot of them on top of your dishes for a flavorful and healthy meal.

6. Avoid sugar and processed foods:
   - Handled food varieties and unreasonable sugar admission can add to aggravation. To support an anti-inflammatory lifestyle, choose whole, unprocessed foods whenever possible.

7. Keep hydrated:
   Keeping hydrated is important for your overall health and can help flush out toxins. Your daily routine should include drinking water, herbal teas, and water that has been infused with cucumber or citrus fruit slices.

8. Eating mindfully:
   - Practice careful eating by focusing on yearning and totality prompts. This may aid in better digestion and prevent overeating.

9. Explore different avenues regarding Different Cooking Methods:

- Investigate steaming, cooking, or sautéing rather than profound broiling. The nutritional value of the ingredients is preserved thanks to these methods.

10. Make your diet unique: - Everybody's body responds contrastingly to food varieties. Take note of how certain foods affect your body and tailor your anti-inflammatory diet to meet your specific requirements.

Keep in mind, a calming diet is definitely not a one-size-fits-all methodology, and it's fundamental to talk with a medical services proficient or an enlisted dietitian to make a customized plan that meets your particular wellbeing objectives and necessities.

Chapter Four

Planning and Preparing Meals

Certainly! Making well-thought-out choices is an important part of implementing an anti-inflammatory diet, which aims to lower body inflammation and improve health as a whole. The following is a discussion of the provided aspects of planning:

Week by week Feast Arranging Strategies:

- Assortment of Bright Vegetables and Fruits:
Consolidate a rainbow of vegetables and natural products wealthy in cell reinforcements. Various tones demonstrate different phytonutrients that have calming properties.

- **Omega-3 Greasy Acids:** Incorporate greasy fish (like salmon, mackerel, or sardines) or plant-based wellsprings of omega-3s (flaxseeds, chia seeds, pecans) to assist with neutralizing aggravation.

- **Entire Grains:** Whole grains like quinoa, brown rice, and oats are full of nutrients and fiber that help maintain a healthy gut and reduce inflammation.

- **Lean Proteins:** Lean proteins like beans, tofu, poultry, and lentils provide essential amino acids without a lot of saturated fat.

- **"Safest Fats:"** Incorporate wellsprings of solid fats like avocados, olive oil, and nuts. These fats support overall health and have anti-inflammatory properties.

<u>**Bunch Cooking for Convenience:**</u>

- Bulk Protein Preparation: Lean proteins like chicken or lentils can be cooked in bulk and used in a variety of dishes throughout the week. This can save time and guarantee you have a protein source promptly accessible.

- **Grains and Legumes:** Cook entire grains and vegetables in bunches and store them for speedy augmentations to servings of mixed greens, bowls, or side dishes. This smoothes out the cooking system during occupied days.

- **Keep portions frozen:** Segment out dinners and freeze them for sometime in the future. This is particularly useful for natively constructed soups, stews, or dishes that can be handily warmed.

-**Pre-cut Vegetables:** Wash, hack, and store vegetables in the cooler for simple access. Because of this, adding them to meals doesn't require much time for preparation.

<u>**Making meals with flavor and balance:**</u>

- **Spices and Spices:** Use spices and flavors like turmeric, ginger, garlic, and cinnamon, which have mitigating properties and add flavor without depending on unreasonable salt.

- **Verdant Greens:** Consolidate mixed greens like kale, spinach, and Swiss chard, which are plentiful in nutrients, minerals, and cancer prevention agents.

- **Fermented Meats**: Incorporate aged food varieties like yogurt, kefir, sauerkraut, or kimchi to advance stomach wellbeing. A sound stomach microbiome is connected to decreased irritation.

Hydration: Remain very much hydrated with water, home grown teas, and mixed water with cuts of leafy foods. Legitimate hydration upholds generally speaking wellbeing and can assist with lessening irritation.

By joining these systems, you can make a balanced and helpful mitigating dinner plan that advances generally speaking wellbeing and prosperity.

Certainly! A calming diet centers around diminishing aggravation in the body by consolidating food sources that are wealthy in cell reinforcements, omega-3 unsaturated fats, and other mitigating compounds. Here are a few hints for productive dinner planning, efficient strategies, and getting ready fixings ahead of time for a calming diet:

Tips for Productive Dinner Arrangement:

1. Feast Planning:

- Plan your dinners for the week, consolidating different mitigating food varieties.

- To make grocery shopping easier, make a shopping list based on your meal plan.

2. Cooking in batches:

- Cook in bigger amounts and store extras for later feasts.

During the week, you can save time and ensure that you always have nutritious meals on hand by batch cooking.

3. One-Container Meals:

- Decide on one-skillet or one-pot recipes to limit cleanup time.

A quick and effective method is to roast vegetables and lean proteins on a single sheet pan.

4. Together, prepare similar ingredients:

- Combine similar ingredients by chopping, slicing, or dicing them. This will simplify your preparation.

Cutting boards and knives don't need to be changed as frequently as they used to.

Techniques for Saving Time

1. Utilize Frozen Foods grown from the ground

- Have a supply of frozen vegetables and fruits on hand so that you can quickly add them to smoothies, stir-fries, or side dishes.

- They hold their health benefits and require insignificant arrangement.

2. Spend money on time-saving devices:

- To cut down on time spent chopping and cooking, use kitchen tools like blenders, food processors, and slow cookers.

- Electric strain cookers can fundamentally decrease cooking times for grains, beans, and stews.

3. Produce that has been pre-washed and cut

- Buy pre-cut or pre-washed leafy foods to save time on arrangement.

Even though it costs a little more, it could be a good way to save time.

4. Cook Once, Eat Twice: - Prepare additional portions and incorporate them into other dishes.

- For instance, barbecued chicken can be utilized in servings of mixed greens, wraps, or as a protein source in different dishes.

<u>Getting ready Fixings Ahead of time:</u>

1. Clean and chop veggies:

- Wash and slash vegetables ahead of time and store them in sealed shut holders.

- It is simpler to incorporate vegetables into meals when they have already been prepared.

2. Pre-cook Grains and Legumes:
- Prepare large quantities of lentils, brown rice, or quinoa in advance and store them in the refrigerator.

These essentials can be quickly incorporated into salads, bowls, or side dishes.

3. Marinate Proteins:
- Marinate proteins (chicken, tofu, fish) ahead of time and store them in the fridge or cooler.
- This lessens cooking time and improves flavor.

4. Make smoothie bundles:
- Place smoothie ingredients, like greens and fruits, in freezer bags before making the smoothie.

For a quick and healthy smoothie in the morning, simply blend the contents with liquid.

By consolidating these tips and procedures, you can smooth out your dinner arrangement cycle and make it more straightforward to follow a calming diet. Preparing and having promptly accessible fixings will add to better dietary patterns and save you time over the long haul.

Chapter Five

Overcoming Obstacles

Certainly! Taking on a calming diet includes pursuing cognizant food decisions to diminish irritation in the body. This can be testing while feasting out or going to get-togethers, where the food choices may not necessarily in every case line up with a mitigating way of life. Here are a few ways to explore these circumstances:

Feasting Out on a Mitigating Diet:

1. Pick Lean Proteins:
   - Settle on barbecued or prepared fish, chicken, or lean meats.
   - Consume proteins derived from plants, such as tofu, beans, and lentils.

2. Embrace Sound Fats: - Choose dishes ready with olive oil, avocado oil, or coconut oil.

- Incorporate omega-3-rich foods like salmon and walnuts.

3. Load Up on Vegetables:

- Choose dishes that include a variety of vibrant, starchy vegetables.

- Think about serving entrees or side dishes with vegetables.

4. Be Aware of Carbohydrates:

- Pick entire grains over refined grains (earthy colored rice, quinoa, entire wheat).

- Limit handled starches and sweet choices.

5. Limit or Avoid Dairy:

- Use almond or coconut milk instead of dairy.

- Eat cheese and yogurt in moderation, or look into alternatives that don't contain dairy.

6. Request Modifications:
   - Feel free to make adjustments to suit your dietary inclinations.
   - Demand sauces and dressings as an afterthought to control segment sizes.

7. Remain Hydrated:
   Keep hydrated and drink a lot of water to support your overall health.
   - Limit sweet beverages and decide on natural teas or water with lemon.

Choosing the Right Restaurant:

1. Research the Menu: - Look into the eatery's menu ahead of time to design your decisions.
   - Pick cafés that offer different new, entire food varieties.

2. Communicate with the Workers:
   - Let your server know if you have any dietary preferences or restrictions.
    - Get some information about fixing replacements or readiness techniques.

3. Control of portions:
   - Share larger dishes and be mindful of portion sizes.
   - Keep away from the impulse to gorge by paying attention to your body's craving prompts.

4. Keep away from Broiled Foods:
   - Decide on barbecued, heated, or steamed choices as opposed to broiled.
    - Seared food sources frequently contain provocative oils.

Methods for Social Events:

1. Include a Dish:
   - Bring a dish that goes well with your anti-inflammatory diet to share.
   - This guarantees you have a sound choice accessible.

2. Impart Dietary Preferences:
   - Provide the host with advance notice of your dietary preferences.
   - If it helps to accommodate your requirements, offer to bring a dish.

3. Eat Beforehand:
   - Have a nutritious feast or tidbit prior to going to a get-together.
   This may assist in reducing hunger and the likelihood of making poor choices.

4. Pick Wisely:
   - Examine all of the options and put whole, unprocessed foods first.

- Fill your plate with vegetables, lean proteins, and solid fats.

5. Limit Liquor and Sweet Drinks:
    - If you drink alcohol at all, do so in moderation.
    - Select water, home grown tea, or other non-improved drinks.

Embracing a calming diet doesn't mean forfeiting social encounters. You can navigate dining out and social gatherings while still giving your health priority by planning ahead, making informed decisions, and communicating your needs.

Chapter Six

Lifestyle and Prolonged Health

Practice and Its Part in Lessening Inflammation:

Irritation is a characteristic reaction of the invulnerable framework to injury or contamination. However, a number of diseases, including diabetes, autoimmune disorders, and cardiovascular problems, are linked to chronic inflammation. In order to control inflammation, regular exercise is very important.

Positive Effect of Exercise:
Normal active work has been reliably connected to a decrease in ongoing irritation. The body's ability to effectively manage inflammation is enhanced by the cascade of physiological responses triggered by exercise.

Mechanisms of Action:
- Regulation of Cytokine: Cytokines, which are the signaling molecules involved in inflammation, are influenced by exercise in both their production and release. With regular exercise, pro-inflammatory cytokines decrease, while anti-inflammatory cytokines increase.

- **Insulin Sensitivity:** The risk of insulin resistance and subsequent inflammation is decreased when insulin sensitivity is improved through exercise.

- **Weight Control:** Keeping a sound load through practice is urgent, as overabundance of muscle to fat ratio, particularly around the stomach region, is related with expanded irritation.

Recommendations

The Amcrican Heart Affiliation suggests no less than 150 minutes of moderate-force practice each week. This can incorporate exercises like lively strolling, running, swimming, or cycling. Additionally, performing strength training exercises at least twice per week aids in overall anti-inflammatory effects.

<u>Selecting the Best Exercises:</u>

Different kinds of exercise have different effects on inflammation. A balanced work-out routine ought to incorporate a blend of oxygen consuming exercises, strength preparing, and adaptability.

Aerobic Exercise:

Exercises that are aerobic or cardiovascular raise breathing and heart rate. These exercises, like running, cycling, and vigorous dance, show critical mitigating impacts. They upgrade flow, advance cardiovascular wellbeing, and add to general prosperity.

Training for Strength:
Constructing and keeping up with bulk through strength preparing practices add to diminished irritation. Opposition preparing further develops insulin responsiveness and metabolic wellbeing, the two of which are critical in overseeing persistent irritation.

Exercises for Flexibility and Balance:
Yoga and tai chi, for example, not only improve flexibility and balance, but they also reduce inflammation. The brain body association in these activities, joined with controlled developments, adds to pressure decrease and in general aggravation control.

Adding movement to your daily routine:

Moving around on a daily basis is essential for maintaining an active and healthy lifestyle, in addition to scheduled workouts. Inflammation levels can be significantly impacted by subtle, consistent changes.

Breaks as a result of prolonged sitting:

Increased inflammation has been linked to prolonged sitting positions. Enjoying short reprieves consistently to stand, stretch, or walk can check the adverse consequences of delayed sitting on the body.

Daily Activities:

Straightforward changes in everyday exercises can add to expanded development. Picking steps rather than lifts, strolling brief distances as opposed to driving, and participating in exercises like planting or house keeping all add to generally speaking active work.

Consistency is Key:

Consistency is critical with regards to development. Consolidating little, sensible changes into everyday schedules is more supportable over the long haul, assisting with keeping a functioning way of life.

<u>Strategies for Stress Management:</u>

Stress is a huge supporter of constant irritation. Overseeing pressure through different procedures can decidedly affect general well being and aggravation levels.

Impact of Persistent Stress:
Cortisol, a hormone associated with the body's "fight or flight" response, is released when chronic stress is present. A compromised immune system and increased inflammation can result from persistent cortisol elevation.

Techniques for Stress Management:

-Profound Breathing: Rehearsing profound, diaphragmatic breathing actuates the parasympathetic sensory system, advancing unwinding and lessening pressure.

- Moderate Muscle Unwinding (PMR):

PMR includes deliberately straining and loosening up various muscle gatherings, advancing physical and mental unwinding.

- Biofeedback: Biofeedback techniques aid in stress reduction by bringing people's awareness and control over physiological functions like heart rate and muscle tension.

Mind-Body Exercises:
Care based pressure decrease (MBSR), contemplation, and directed symbolism are instances of brain body rehearses that have shown viability in pressure decrease. These practices lighten pressure as well as add to a decrease in provocative markers.

<u>**The Effect of Weight on Inflammation:**</u>

Understanding the multifaceted connection among stress and irritation is essential in embracing compelling procedures to oversee the two parts of wellbeing.

Hormonal Reaction to Stress:
The body's pressure reaction includes the arrival of cortisol and adrenaline. While these chemicals are fundamental for endurance in intense pressure circumstances, ongoing pressure can prompt supported height of cortisol levels, adding to irritation.

Stress's effect on behavior:
Constant pressure frequently prompts unfortunate survival techniques, like unfortunate dietary decisions, inactive way of behaving, and upset rest. These actions make inflammation get worse even more, opening up a vicious cycle that can lead to a variety of health problems.

Individual Variability:
Different people respond differently to
stress. Individual variation in stress
responses and their impact on inflammation
are influenced by genetic, environmental,
and psychological factors.

Care and Unwinding Practices:

Care and unwinding rehearses center
around developing a present-second
mindfulness and advancing mental and
profound prosperity, which, thus, can
emphatically impact irritation.

Interventions Based on Mindfulness:
- MBSR: Mindfulness-based stress
reduction programs teach people to focus on
the present moment, which helps them deal
with stress and the inflammation it causes.

- Eating in a Mindful Way: The sensory experience of eating, such as taste and texture, can help people choose healthier foods and improve digestion, thereby reducing inflammation.

Yoga and Tai Chi:

Yoga and judo join actual stances, controlled breathing, and reflection. In addition to improving flexibility and balance, these practices also aid in stress reduction and have anti-inflammatory effects.

Sleep Quality:

Care practices can work on the nature of rest, and satisfactory rest is vital for generally speaking wellbeing and irritation control. Unfortunate rest designs are related with expanded irritation and increased pressure reactions.

In conclusion, adopting an anti-inflammatory diet is a holistic approach to health that should be complemented by regular exercise, the selection of the right exercises, consistent daily movement, stress management strategies, an understanding of the impact of stress on inflammation, and the incorporation of mindfulness and relaxation practices. Including these components in a comprehensive lifestyle plan can have a significant and beneficial effect on lowering chronic inflammation and improving well-being as a whole.

Conclusion

Certainly! We should examine the proposed "End" segment of your "Calming Diet Cookbook for Fledglings 2024."

Recognizing Achievements

The conclusion is an opportunity to encourage and celebrate the reader's journey toward adopting an anti-inflammatory lifestyle.

Celebrating Your Anti-Inflammatory Journey

Recognize the endeavors they have made and the positive changes they've integrated into their everyday daily schedule. This segment ought to accentuate that each little step counts and that advancement, regardless of how gradual, merits celebrating.

Moving Forward with a Healthier Lifestyle

Shows readers how to move from the cookbook to a healthier lifestyle that lasts. Urge them to keep investigating new recipes, exploring different avenues regarding flavors, and remaining drawn in with the standards of the mitigating diet. Build up the possibility that this isn't simply a transient eating regimen however a drawn out obligation to generally wellbeing and prosperity.

Final Reflection

Reflecting on Progress

Ask readers to consider how far they have come since beginning the anti-inflammatory diet. Encourage them to reflect on the changes in their mood, energy, and overall well-being. Allow readers to evaluate the positive effects of their dietary choices by providing prompts for self-reflection.

Keeping Motivated

Provide readers with tips for staying motivated to continue their anti-inflammatory journey. This could incorporate putting forth new objectives, investigating extra assets, or interfacing with a strong local area. Share examples of overcoming adversity or tributes from people who have encountered huge enhancements in their wellbeing by following a mitigating way of life.

Future Advances

Past the Cookbook

Give direction on what perusers can investigate past the cookbook. This could remember suggesting further pursuits for mitigating nourishment, recommending important narratives, or empowering cooperation in cooking classes or studios. Enable perusers to keep growing their insight and refining their culinary abilities.

Integrating Way of life Changes

Feature the interconnected idea of way of life factors, like pressure on the board and standard actual work, related to the calming diet. Inspire readers to investigate additional healthy lifestyle choices that complement their diets.

Offering Thanks

Offer thanks to the perusers for picking your cookbook and making strides towards a better life. Reassure them that they have the knowledge and tools they need to keep making good choices and thank them for entrusting you with their journey.

Source of inspiration

Sharing Achievement

Urge perusers to share their examples of overcoming adversity, criticism, and most loved recipes from the cookbook. Make a space, whether through a devoted site, online entertainment, or a local area gathering, where users can interface, move one another, and share their mitigating encounters.

You are providing readers with a sense of accomplishment, motivation, and a road map for the ongoing journey toward better health through the anti-inflammatory diet's principles by carefully crafting the conclusion. This end ought to leave perusers feeling enabled and enlivened to keep going with good decisions for their prosperity.

Appendix

Certainly! The "Index" part of your "Mitigating Diet Cookbook for Novices 2024" fills in as a strengthening asset for perusers, offering extra data, devices, and references that supplement the substance of the principal sections. An overview of what might go in the appendix is as follows:

Extra Assets

Suggested Perusing
Order a rundown of books, articles, and examination papers connected with mitigating nourishment, wellbeing, and sound living. Sort them according to the particular subjects covered in your cookbook. Give a concise portrayal of every asset to direct perusers in choosing materials that line up with their inclinations and objectives.

Online Platforms and Communities

Provide links to reputable websites, blogs, and online communities where readers can find ongoing support, expert guidance, and community involvement in relation to the anti-inflammatory lifestyle. This could incorporate gatherings, web-based entertainment gatherings, and sites of wellbeing and sustenance experts.

Glossary of Terms

Key Fixings
Order a glossary of key fixings utilized in the cookbook, particularly those that may be less natural to fledglings. Define terms like turmeric, quinoa, and specific spices and herbs that can reduce inflammation. Remember data for the medical advantages of every fixing.

Terms Used in Nutrition

Define and discuss terms that are frequently used in relation to nutrition and the anti-inflammatory diet. This could incorporate terms like cancer prevention agents, omega-3 unsaturated fats, and polyphenols. Make it clear how these concepts relate to the anti-inflammatory diet's overall objectives.

Estimation Changes

Metric to Majestic Changes

Give a change graph to perusers who might be more acquainted with metric or supreme estimations. Incorporate changes for normal cooking units like grams to ounces, liters to cups, and Celsius to Fahrenheit. This can assist with guaranteeing precision and consistency while following recipes.

Portion Sizes and Equivalents

Outline common food item portion sizes and equivalents. In order to keep a healthy and balanced diet, this information can help readers comprehend and control their food intake.

Recipe Record

Sequential Posting
Make a sequential record of the multitude of recipes highlighted in the cookbook. Incorporate page numbers for simple reference. This permits perusers to find and return to their #1 recipe rapidly.

Categorized Index
Organize the recipes by category (for example, breakfast, lunch, dinner, and snacks) to make it easier for readers to find recipes that meet their dietary requirements and preferences.

Clear Recipe Pages

Individual Recipe Diary
Incorporate a couple of clear pages where users can write down their own number one recipes or changes to the ones given in the cookbook. This fills in as a space for personalization and imagination.

Conclusion

Closing Notes At the end of the appendix, thank the readers once more and urge them to make the most of the resources provided. Reiterate your support for their efforts to improve their health and provide any additional guidance or advice for making effective use of the appendix.

The reference section fills in as a significant asset for users looking for more top to bottom data, explanation, and association of the substance introduced in the fundamental parts of the cookbook. It provides a comprehensive guide for individuals who are committed to adopting and maintaining an anti-inflammatory lifestyle in addition to enhancing the overall user experience.